MW00872490

Contents

Introduction

The term "gastritis" refers to any of a number of different digestive health conditions in which the lining of the stomach becomes inflamed. Gastritis can affect just about anyone and can be caused by many different factors. One of the most common forms of gastritis is caused by medication in particular, non-steroidal anti-inflammatory drugs(NSAIDs). These widely used painkillers, which include ibuprofen (Advil, Motrin) and naproxen (Aleve), are known to affect the stomach and lead to irritation and swelling if taken on a routine basis.Older people or those with weakened immune systems are at a greater risk of developing gastritis. Some people may have genetic abnormalities that predispose them to developing gastritis. Those who take NSAIDs consistently to treat chronic conditions like arthritis or pain should be aware of their risk of developing gastritis and talk to their doctors about protecting their stomachs.Besides smokers and heavy drinkers, others at risk of getting gastritis include those who drink acidic beverages (like coffee) and are under constant stress (which produces lots of gastric acid).

Depending on the cause of the inflammation, gastritis can be classified as chronic or acute, with the former being characterised by long term symptoms such as loss of appetite or nausea, and the latter by short term, severe symptoms lasting a day or two. Gastritis is a common condition, affecting roughly one in five Australians, typically between the ages of 15 and 50. Some people with the condition don't display any identifiable symptoms.Some forms of gastritis are significantly less common but can have much more severe symptoms. Erosive gastritis doesn't typically cause much in the way of inflammation but can lead to bleeding or ulcers in the stomach. Chronic atrophic gastritis, a rare form of gastritis usually caused by the helicobacter pylori (H. pylori) bacteria is characterised by destruction of the mucosal barrier that protects the stomach and atrophy of cells in the lining of the stomach and can increase the risk of a person developing stomach cancer. Pernicious anaemia (which is another gastric disorder), may be associated with chronic, atrophic gastritis.

Gastritis

Your stomach lining has an important job. It makes acid and enzymes that help break down food so you can extract the nutrients you need. The lining also protects itself from acid damage by secreting mucus. But sometimes the lining gets inflamed and starts making less acid, enzymes and mucus. This type of inflammation is called gastritis, and it can cause long-term problems.

Some people think they have gastritis when they have pain or an uncomfortable feeling in their upper stomach. But many other conditions can cause these symptoms. Gastritis can sometimes lead to pain, nausea and vomiting. But it often has no symptoms at all. If left untreated, though, some types of gastritis can lead to ulcers (sores in the stomach lining) or even stomach cancer.

People used to think gastritis and ulcers were caused by stress and spicy foods. But research studies show that bacteria called Helicobacter pylori are often to blame. Usually, these bacteria cause no symptoms. In the United States, 20% to 50% of the population may be infected with H. pylori.

H. pylori breaks down the inner protective coating in some people's stomachs and causes inflammation. I tell people H. pylori is like having termites in your stomach. You usually don't know you have termites until someone tells you, and you ignore it at your own risk. H. pylori can spread by passing from person to person or through contaminated food or water. Infections can be treated with bacteria-killing drugs called antibiotics.

One type of gastritis, called erosive gastritis, wears away the stomach lining. The most common cause of erosive gastritis is long-term use of medications called non-steroidal anti-inflammatory drugs. These include aspirin and ibuprofen. When you stop taking the drugs, the condition usually goes away. Doctors might also recommend reducing the dose or switching to another class of pain medication.

Less common causes of gastritis include certain digestive disorders (such as Crohn's disease) and autoimmune disorders, in which the body's protective immune cells mistakenly attack healthy cells in the stomach lining.

Gastritis can be diagnosed with an endoscope, a thin tube with a tiny camera on the end, which is inserted through the patient's mouth or nose and into the stomach. The doctor will look at the stomach lining and may also remove some tissue samples for testing.Treatment will depend on the type of gastritis you have.

Although stress and spicy foods don't cause gastritis and ulcers, they can make symptoms worse. Milk might provide brief relief, but it also increases stomach acid, which can worsen symptoms. Your doctor may recommend taking antacids or other drugs to reduce acid in the stomach.

Medical definition of gastritis

Gastritis is inflammation of the stomach lining. There are two types of gastritis, acute and chronic.

signs and symptoms of gastritis

Some people with gastritis may not have any symptoms; however, both acute and chronic gastritis may have symptoms and signs of abdominal pain, nausea, vomiting, and occasionally, belching, bloating, loss of appetite and indigestion.

What causes gastritis?

A bacterium called Helicobacter pylori or H. pylori, and nonsteroidal anti-inflammatory drugs (NSAIDs) are the two main causes of gastritis; however, there are many other causes of the condition, for example, infectious agents, autoimmune problems, diseases like Crohn's disease, sarcoidosis, and isolated granulomatosis gastritis.

How do you know if you have gastritis?

Gastritis can be diagnosed by the your symptoms and history (for example, NSAID and/or alcohol consumption), or by breath, blood, stool, immunological, and biopsy tests to detect H. pylori, and other tests like endoscopy or radiologic studies demonstrate mucosal changes.

What is the treatment for gastritis?

The treatment for gastritis varies according to the cause. Other less common causes may be treated similarly, but do not treat the underlying cause.

Is there a diet for gastritis?

Gastritis symptoms can be aggravated by chemical irritants that cause or aggravate the symptoms of gastritis should be reduced or stopped all together. For example, stop smoking cigarettes, avoid drinking excessive amounts of alcohol, avoid caffeinated, decaffeinated, and carbonated drinks; and fruit juices that contain citric acid, for example, grapefruit, orange, pineapple, etc., and avoid high-fat foods.

There is no gastritis diet, however, the growth of H. pylori may be stopped by a diet rich in fiber, and foods that contain flavonoids, for example, certain teas, onions, garlic, berries, celery, kale, broccoli, parsley, thyme, foods with soy, and legumes, for example, lentils, kidney, black, soy, pinto, and navy beans.

What home remedies help reduce symptoms of gastritis?

Home remedies may help reduce gastritis symptoms, but usually does not treat the underlying cause of the condition.

How long does it take for gastritis to go away?

People with acute gastritis usually recover completely with no complications. However, chronic gastritis may have a range of outcomes from good (early treatment) to poor if serious complications develop. Rarely, complications can occur from acute gastritis.

Complications from chronic gastritis include peptic ulcer, bleeding ulcers, anemia, gastric cancers, MALT lymphoma, renal problems, strictures, bowel obstruction, or even death.

If underlying causes of gastritis (for example, alcohol, or NSAIDs usage) are treated or not used, gastritis also may be prevented.

Can gastritis be cured?

Gastritis may be cured if the underlying cause(s) is cured.

How can you prevent gastritis?

Since gastritis is infections and can you can avoid it by practicing good hand washing techniques, for example, wash the hands thoroughly and frequently. To reduce the risk of gastritis avoid situations where you are exposed to chemicals, radiation, or toxins.

What is gastritis

Gastritis is inflammation of the lining of the stomach. Unfortunately, the term "gastritis" has been misused to include many different upper abdominal problems, but true gastritis refers to the stomach lining (gastric mucosa) that is inflamed. All or part of the gastric mucosa may be involved. Gastritis may be classified as acute or chronic.Acute gastritis maybe characterized as erosive (damaged areas where mucosal cells are disrupted or missing) and nonerosive. Chronic gastritis is determined by histopathology (appearance of the gastric mucosa) with symptoms lasting a long time. There is no widely accepted classification system although some have been proposed.

This information will focus on true gastritis. Gastritis has many causes, but most causes result in similar symptoms. This has leads to some confusion and is the reason why many health-care professionals now consider the term "gastritis" as a non-specific description of a cluster of symptoms.

Acute gastritis lasts for about 2-10 days. If chronic gastritis is not treated, it may last from weeks to years.

Symptoms of gastritis

Many people with gastritis do not have symptoms. The condition is diagnosed only when samples of the stomach mucosa are examined for other suspected diseases. However, when gastritis symptoms occur, the most common symptoms include abdominal pain (intermittent or constant burning, gripping or gnawing pain), nausea and vomiting, diarrhea, loss of appetite, bloating, burping, and belching.

Gastritis symptoms come and go over time, especially with chronic gastritis. Indigestion (dyspepsia) is another term that encompasses this cluster of symptoms. Symptoms of severe gastritis may include, vomiting blood, blood in the stool, and anemia

Can you drink alcohol and eat any foods with gastritis

Foods and other substances that should be avoided to reduce or prevent gastritis symptoms include, alcohol, spicy, fatty, and fried foods. Moreover, anything that might be toxic or irritating to the stomach should also be avoided (for example cigarette smoking, acidic drinks like coffee, garlic powder, chili powder, peppers and tomato products).

Foods that may stop H. pylori growth and relieve gastritis symptoms include:

- Teas (green and white in particular)
- Yogurt
- Peppermint
- Wheat bran
- Carrot juice
- Coconut water
- Green leafy vegetables
- Onions
- Garlic
- Apples
- Fresh fruits and berries
- Celery
- Cranberry juice
- Kale

- Broccoli
- Scallions
- Parsley
- Thyme
- Soybeans
- Soy foods
- Legumes (beans, peas, and lentils)

Although these home remedies may help reduce or soothe symptoms, home remedies seldom treat the underlying causes of gastritis.

Causes of gastritis

A major cause of both acute and chronic gastritis is infection of the stomach mucosa by a bacterial species named Helicobacter pylori. Usually, this bacterium first infects the stomach antrum (stomach mucosa without acid-producing cells) acutely and may progress to infect most or all of the stomach's mucosa over time (chronic gastritis) and remain there for years. This infection generates an initial strong inflammatory response and eventually, a long-term chronic inflammation with intestinal cell changes may develop. Another major cause of acute and chronic gastritis is the use (and overuse) of nonsteroidal anti-inflammatory drugs (NSAIDs).

However, there are many other causes of gastritis; the following is a list of common causes of both acute and chronic gastritis; chronic gastritis may occur with repeated or continual presence of most of these causes:

- Bacterial, viral and parasitic infections
- Certain drugs (cocaine)
- Alcoholic disease (drinking excessive amounts of alcohol)
- Bile reflux
- Fungal infections
- Allergic reactions
- Autoimmune reactions
- Stress reaction
- Radiation
- Certain food poisonings (infectious and chemical)

- Trauma

In general, infectious agents, especially Helicobacter pylori, and NSAIDs are responsible for the majority of people with gastritis.

How do you know if you have gastritis

Gastritis is diagnosed based on the patient's symptoms and history of a previous diagnosis and treatment of gastritis, alcohol consumption, and use of NSAIDs. Definitive diagnosis of gastritis is made by identifying the underlying cause of the gastric mucosal inflammation and/or by tissue (gastric) biopsy. For example, the major infective cause of gastritis is Helicobacter pylori (H. pylori). This bacterium can be detected by breath, blood, stool, immunological and biopsy tests. Although the bacterium can be cultured from the patient, this is seldom attempted. Other pathogens can be identified using culture, stool, and immunological tests.

Biopsy of the stomach mucosa, done during endoscopy examinations, is often used in patients to identify the causes of chronic gastritis and may allow visualization of mucosal erosions and other stomach mucosal changes. Abdominal X-rays or barium studies (upper or lower) may demonstrate the presence of thickened mucosa and folds that are signs of inflammation in the stomach.

Your doctor can help determine which tests should be done, including ancillary tests that may help identify other causes of the non-specific symptoms commonly found with gastritis.

Treatment of Gastritis

Treatment of gastritis depends on the specific cause. Acute gastritis caused by nonsteroidal anti-inflammatory drugs or alcohol may be relieved by stopping use of those substances.

Medications used to treat gastritis include:

1. Antibiotic medications to kill H. pylori.For H. pylori in your digestive tract, your doctor may recommend a combination of antibiotics, such as

clarithromycin (Biaxin) and amoxicillin (Amoxil, Augmentin, others) or metronidazole (Flagyl), to kill the bacterium.Be sure to take the full antibiotic prescription, usually for seven to 14 days.

2. Medications that block acid production and promote healing. Proton pump inhibitors reduce acid by blocking the action of the parts of cells that produce acid. These drugs include the prescription and over-the-counter medications omeprazole (Prilosec), lansoprazole (Prevacid), rabeprazole (Aciphex), esomeprazole (Nexium), dexlansoprazole (Dexilant) and pantoprazole (Protonix).
3. Long-term use of proton pump inhibitors, particularly at high doses, may increase your risk of hip, wrist and spine fractures. Ask your doctor whether a calcium supplement may reduce this risk.
4. Medications to reduce acid production. Acid blockers also called histamine (H-2) blockers reduce the amount of acid released into your

digestive tract, which relieves gastritis pain and encourages healing. Available by prescription or over-the-counter, acid blockers include famotidine (Pepcid), cimetidine (Tagamet HB) and nizatidine (Axid AR).

5. Antacids that neutralize stomach acid. Your doctor may include an antacid in your drug regimen. Antacids neutralize existing stomach acid and can provide rapid pain relief. Side effects can include constipation or diarrhea, depending on the main ingredients.

Lifestyle and home remedies

You may find some relief from signs and symptoms if you:

- Eat smaller, more-frequent meals.If you experience frequent indigestion, eat smaller meals more often to help ease the effects of stomach acid.
- Avoid irritating foods. Avoid foods that irritate your stomach, especially those that are spicy, acidic, fried or fatty.

- Avoid alcohol. Alcohol can irritate the mucous lining of your stomach.
- Consider switching pain relievers. If you use pain relievers that increase your risk of gastritis, ask your doctor whether acetaminophen (Tylenol, others) may be an option for you.This medication is less likely to aggravate your stomach problem.

Preparing for your appointment

Start by making an appointment with your family doctor or a general practitioner. If your doctor suspects gastritis, you may be referred to a specialist in digestive disorders (gastroenterologist).

What you can do

- Be aware of pre-appointment restrictions. When you make the appointment, ask if there's anything you need to do in advance, such as restrict your diet.
- Write down symptoms you're experiencing, including any that may seem unrelated to the reason for which you scheduled the appointment.

- Write down key personal information, including major stresses or recent life changes.
- Make a list of all medications, vitamins or supplements you're taking.
- Consider taking someone along. Someone who accompanies you may remember something that you missed or forgot.
- Write down questions to ask your doctor.

Preparing a list of questions will help you make the most of your time with your doctor. For gastritis, some basic questions to ask your doctor include:

- What is likely causing my symptoms or condition?
- Could any of my medications be causing my condition?
- What are other possible causes for my symptoms or condition?
- What tests do I need?
- Is my condition likely temporary or chronic?
- What is the best course of action?

- What are alternatives to the primary approach you're suggesting?
- I have other health conditions. How can I best manage them together?
- Are there restrictions that I need to follow?
- Should I see a specialist?
- Is there a generic alternative to the medicine you're prescribing?
- Are there brochures or other printed material I can take?What websites do you recommend?
- What will determine whether I should schedule a follow-up visit?

Don't hesitate to ask other questions.

What to expect from your doctor

Your doctor is likely to ask you a number of questions, including:

- What are your symptoms?
- How severe are your symptoms? Would you describe your stomach pain as mildly uncomfortable or burning?

- Have your symptoms been continuous or occasional?
- Does anything, such as eating certain foods, seem to worsen your symptoms?
- Does anything, such as eating certain foods or taking antacids, seem to improve your symptoms?
- Do you experience any nausea or vomiting?
- Have you recently lost weight?
- How often do you take pain relievers, such as aspirin, ibuprofen or naproxen?
- How often do you drink alcohol, and how much do you drink?
- How would you rate your stress level?
- Have you noticed any black stools or blood in your stool?
- Have you ever had an ulcer?

Treating gastritis and gastropathy

Your doctor will recommend treatments based on the type of gastritis or gastropathy you have and its cause. Treating gastritis and gastropathy can improve symptoms, if present, and lower your chance of complications.

H. pylori gastritis

Doctors treat Helicobacter pylori (H. pylori) gastritis with a combination of medicines to kill

H. pylori bacteria. These medicines most often include

- two or more antibiotics NIH external link
- a proton pump inhibitor (PPI) NIH external link
- in some cases, bismuth subsalicylate NIH external link

Your doctor may avoid prescribing antibiotics you've taken in the past because the H. pylori bacteria may have developed antibiotic resistance NIH external link to those antibiotics.

If you are given medicines, take all doses exactly as your doctor prescribes. If you stop taking your medicine early, some bacteria may survive and reinfect you. In other words, H. pylori bacteria may develop antibiotic resistance.

To find out if medicines have worked, your health care professional may recommend testing you for H. pylori at least 4 weeks after you've finished taking medicines.4 If you still have an H. pylori infection, your doctor may prescribe a different combination of antibiotics and other medicines to treat the infection. Making sure that all of the H. pylori bacteria have been killed is important to prevent further complications of the infection.

Reactive gastropathy

If long-term use of nonsteroidal anti-inflammatory drugs (NSAIDs) leads to reactive gastropathy, your doctor may recommend that you stop taking NSAIDs, take a lower dose, or take a different medicine for pain. Doctors may also recommend taking a PPI along with NSAIDs to prevent or treat reactive gastropathy and its possible complications.

If bile reflux is causing reactive gastropathy, doctors may prescribe ursodiol NIH external link, a medicine that contains bile acids and can help heal the stomach lining, or surgery to stop flow of bile into the stomach.

Autoimmune gastritis

If you have autoimmune gastritis, your doctor may recommend iron NIH external link, folic acid NIH external link, and vitamin B12 NIH external link supplements to prevent pernicious anemia. If autoimmune gastritis leads to pernicious anemia NIH external link, doctors may recommend vitamin B12 injections to treat this condition.

For safety reasons, talk with your doctor before using dietary supplements, such as vitamins, or any complementary or alternative NIH external link medicines or medical practices.

Acute erosive gastropathy

For patients with severe injuries or critical illness, doctors may prescribe medicines that reduce stomach acid such as PPIs, H2 blockers NIH external link, or sucralfate (Carafate) NIH external link to prevent or treat stress gastritis.

If an irritating substance is causing acute erosive gastropathy, treatment includes removing contact with the substance. Doctors may also prescribe PPIs or H2 blockers to reduce stomach acid.

If acute erosive gastropathy causes severe bleeding in the stomach, doctors may treat the bleeding during upper GI endoscopy or with surgery in severe cases.

What OTC and prescription medications treat gastritis

Treating the underlying cause of gastritis is the most effective way to reduce or resolve gastritis symptoms. For example, if the cause of gastritis is H. pylori, then treatment with appropriate antibiotics (usually a combination of amoxicillin and clarithromycin [Biaxin, Biaxin XL] plus bismuth subsalicylate [Pepto-Bismol]) should be effective to provide relief from symptoms.

If NSAIDs are the cause, then stopping the drug should be effective.

Other treatments often are used in addition to those that treat the specific cause of gastritis, many of which are over-the-counter or OTC, may reduce or stop symptoms of gastritis and allow gastric mucosal healing to begin regardless of the underlying cause. These medications include

- antacids (Maalox , Rolaids, and Alka-Seltzer),
- histamine (H2) blockers (famotidine [Pepcid AC], ranitidine [Zantac 75]), and
- PPI's or proton pump inhibitors (omeprazole [Prilosec], pantoprazole [Protonix], esomeprazole [Nexium]).

They all function by different mechanisms to reduce acid in the stomach but usually do not treat the underlying cause of gastritis.

What is the best treatment for gastritis

Treatments for gastritis vary and depend on successful treatments of its underlying cause(s). The most common treatments are over-the-counter (OTC) and prescription medications for symptom relief.

A diet that avoids hot, fried and/or spicy foods, alcohol drinking, or eating items you may be allergic to is another good way to both treat and reduce the risk of gastritis.

Home remedies relieve symptoms of gastritis

Usually, home remedies do not treat the underlying cause of gastritis.

Diet for gastritis

There are general recommendations about what foods and drinks that you should consume to help reduce and relieve symptoms of gastritis. If underlying causes are not treated (for example, severe H. pylori infection, eating spicy foods and/or alcohol consumption), diet changes may result in little or no change in gastritis symptoms.

Most people that get gastritis have few or short-term symptoms, and recover completely and are cured of the condition. Those people with underlying causes that are appropriately treated often recover completely. The prognosis of individuals with chronic disease and those who develop serious complications like bleeding ulcers, obstruction, and cancer .

The complications of gastritis may occur over time, especially if gastritis becomes chronic and the underlying causes are not treated. Complications of gastritis may include, peptic ulcer, bleeding ulcers, erosive stomach lining (the stomach tissue wears away), anemia, gastric cancers, MALT lymphoma, gastric scarring and strictures with outlet obstruction, dehydration, kidney problems, and death.

If the underlying cause of gastritis is preventable, then gastritis can be prevented and people can get gastritis relief.

- Don't drink alcohol, take NSAIDs, and quit smoking if they trigger gastritis.
- Avoid situations where chemicals, radiation or some toxin ingestion could be.

It may be more difficult to prevent some infectious causes of gastritis, but proper hygiene, hand washing, and eating and drinking only adequately cleaned or treated foods and fluids are healthy ways to decrease your risk of getting gastritis from infectious agents.

Gastritis Diet

One of the first changes you can make is following a gastritis diet, which can help you manage your symptoms and may even help prevent gastritis. The basic tenet of the gastritis diet is to avoid acidic, spicy foods in favor of low-acid, low sugar foods.

Benefits

As with many health conditions, there are certain risk factors that make a person more likely to develop gastritis. Some of these factors, such as genetics, are not something you have control over. Others, like lifestyle factors, are modifiable.

Diet is one area where you may feel motivated to make changes even before you have been diagnosed with gastritis. The symptoms of the condition may make you feel sick after eating certain foods, which you'll naturally want to avoid.

Even if there aren't specific meals that seem to irritate your stomach, having chronic stomach problems will likely make you more aware of what you eat when you eat, and how much you eat. Following a gastritis diet can help you manage symptoms and may even help you avoid developing the condition if you have risk factors.

If you have been diagnosed with gastritis, paying attention to what you eat can help keep the condition from getting worse. The complications of gastritis can lead to other health problems. For example, stomach bleeding can cause low levels of red blood cells (anemia). If the stomach lining is weakened over time (atrophy) it may increase your risk of developing stomach cancer.

How It Works

If you have gastritis, there are several kinds of treatment your doctor might want you to try, but they'll likely start by having you try making some changes to your diet.

When the lining is inflamed, it can't produce enough of the gastric juices needed for digestion. It also isn't making the mucus that protects it from the stomach acid, which can further damage the tissue.

The broad goal of a gastric diet is to reduce inflammation. There are general recommendations you can start with, such as avoiding foods and drinks frequently linked to stomach irritation (like coffee and acidic fruit). From there you can customize a gastritis diet to suit your individual needs and preferences.

For example, some foods that are typically avoided on the gastritis diet might not bother you as long as you stick to small portions or only have them occasionally. Alternatively, food on the approved list might make your symptoms worse, fail to fit in with your overall dietary needs and preferences or be off-limits for you due to a medical reason (such as a food allergy).

It will be helpful to work with your doctor and other health professionals, such as a registered dietician or nutritionist, to assemble a gastritis diet plan that works best for you.

Duration

Gastritis can be a temporary condition or a chronic one. The length of time you'll need to stick to a gastritis diet will depend on many different factors, such as the symptoms you're having, how long you've had them, the cause of your stomach inflammation, and the other treatments your doctor has prescribed.

In some cases, simply removing a specific trigger is enough to improve your gastritis symptoms. For example, if you have been taking ibuprofen or other over-the-counter pain relievers (NSAIDs) and have gastritis, it may get better if you stop taking these medications.

If you have gastritis due to another health condition, you may need a more long-term strategy for managing your symptoms. The choices you make about your diet will likely be among the more permanent changes you make.

If you are prone to stomach irritation, you may find avoiding caffeine and spicy meals to be key for preventing symptoms. If you only experience symptoms occasionally or they are mild, you might be able to deviate from your gastritis diet once in a while, but you will want to check with your doctor first.

What to Eat

Compliant

- Beans and legumes (as tolerated)
- Eggs, egg whites, or egg substitutes (not fried)
- Seafood, shellfish (not fried)
- Honey
- Low-acid vegetables (cucumber, white potato, carrots)
- Low-sugar, low-acid fruit (pumpkin, blueberries, strawberries, apples)
- Mild, low-salt cheese
- Oats, barley
- Peppermint, ginger, turmeric
- Plain, low-fat yogurt
- Probiotic-rich foods (sauerkraut, kimchi, kombucha)
- Rice
- Skinless lean poultry (chicken, turkey)

- Whole grain bread and pasta

Non-Compliant

- Acidic fruits (citrus) and vegetables (onion)
- Alcohol
- Chocolate
- Coffee and Tea
- Corn and products made with corn (pasta, bread)
- Dairy products
- Energy drinks
- Fatty/greasy food, fast food, spicy food
- Fried or hard-boiled eggs
- Garlic (small amounts as tolerated)
- Ice cream, cakes, and pastries, baked goods
- Marinades, salsa, mayonnaise, creamy sauces
- Nuts and nut butter (small amounts may be tolerated)
- Potato chips, packaged snacks
- Processed meat (sausage, hot dogs), lunch meat
- Red meat, duck, goose

- Refined grains, fresh bread, pasta made with refined flour
- Smoked meats
- Soda, carbonated beverages
- Spices, herbs, seasonings (especially black pepper)
- Tomato and tomato products (juice, paste, sauce)

Fruits and vegetables: Produce that is very acidic, especially citrus fruit and tomatoes, are best avoided if you have gastritis. Vegetables used to add spice or a lot of flavors, such as onions, can also be hard to tolerate if you have stomach irritation.

Instead, choose low-acid or more neutral (alkaline) fruits and veggies—preferably those that are good sources of fiber such as apples, berries, pumpkin, and carrots.

Grains: For the most part you'll want to choose whole grain bread, brown rice, pasta, and other grains. However, if you are having gastritis symptoms that are making it harder for you to eat, plain white rice or white potato can be easier to digest.

Oats, barley, and quinoa are other nutritious options. If you do not eat wheat, avoid pasta alternatives or bread made from corn, which is not approved for a gastritis diet.

Dairy: You'll want to avoid full-fat dairy products, but low-fat yogurt that's also low in sugar and packed with probiotics can be a healthy addition to a gastritis diet. Some hard cheeses that are low in salt may be tolerated in small portions. You'll want to avoid any sauces, fillings, or puddings made with rich, heavy cream.

Protein: Eggs, egg whites, and egg substitutes can be an excellent source of protein. However, you will want to prepare them soft-boiled, poached, or scrambled rather than fried. Avoid pairing them with salty, processed, breakfast meat like sausage or ham, refrain from adding butter or milk, and avoid seasoning (even black pepper).

Red meat is not approved, but you may choose from lean cuts of turkey or chicken and some seafood (as long as it isn't fried).

Nuts and nut butter, as well as beans and legumes, can be high in fat but they are versatile sources of protein to include in your diet. Start with smaller portions (without added sugar) and see what you are able to tolerate.

Desserts: Any food that is high in fat and sugar should be avoided on the gastritis diet. Baked goods, pastries, and ice cream or puddings tend to be rich and can irritate an inflamed stomach (especially if they are made with dairy). Chocolate is also not approved.

Beverages: Some people with mild gastritis can tolerate weak tea or coffee with a splash of low-fat milk or non-dairy creamer. Honey can also be added to tea. In general, though, these beverages are very acidic and not approved for a gastritis diet.

Cold drinks with a lot of sugar, such as soda and energy drinks, are also not approved. Acidic juices (such as orange juice or other citrus fruit, as well as tomato juice) are not approved. Some fruit juice may be OK, but choose varieties that are low in sugar.

Avoid alcoholic beverages, including wine, beer, and cocktails. If you drink alcohol, your doctor will likely advise you to stop if you have gastritis.

Recommended Timing

When your digestive system is under stress or not working optimally, the amount of food you eat and how long you go between meals may contribute to irritation.

If you are prone to having an upset stomach due to gastritis, you may find it helpful to change the timing of your meals and snacks. Try eating smaller meals more frequently throughout the day as opposed to sitting down to three larger ones.

If you don't feel as satisfied when eating less at each meal, add a couple of healthy snacks throughout the day.

Modifications

If you have other health conditions or dietary needs, you may need to adjust the gastritis diet. Gastritis can be caused by other chronic medical conditions, be linked to using certain medications, or be worsened by lifestyle factors—some of which you may be able to change.

You may already follow a particular diet to manage a health condition or avoid food allergens, or you may have specific dietary preferences. You may already be avoiding certain foods that would not be approved for a gastritis diet. For example, if you are lactose intolerant, you are likely already limiting or avoiding dairy products.

If you have celiac disease and need to avoid gluten and wheat, you may need to be careful about the gluten-free alternatives you choose. Some popular options, such as pasta made from corn, are not suitable for a gastritis diet.

At certain times in your life, your dietary needs may change. This is especially true if you are pregnant or breastfeeding. During this time, your nutrition needs will be increased. At the same time, you may be more likely to have gastrointestinal symptoms (both from gastritis if you have it and from other changes happening in your body).

To make sure you are getting enough nourishment and keeping your symptoms under control, you may need to be more flexible with your diet. Let your body be your guide. Some foods that didn't bother you before might start to put you off. You may also "crave" certain foods.

Other health conditions, such as type 2 diabetes, may be influenced by your diet. While a gastritis diet advises you to avoid sugar if you have diabetes and experience an episode of low blood sugar (hypoglycemia) your doctor will likely have you eat something sweet or take a glucose tablet.

If you are managing one or more medical conditions that are affected by what you eat, make sure you ask your doctor about how to best prioritize your dietary needs. Your doctor, dietitian, or nutritionist can help you make sure you are effectively managing your gastritis symptoms and eating a diet that provides the energy and nutrition you need to support your whole-body health.

Cooking Tips

The most important thing to keep in mind when you're preparing or choosing food on a gastritis diet is steering clear of any food that is fried, greasy, fatty, or very sweet and rich. Most notably, these guidelines rule out fast food, but even common preparations or styles of cooking you may be used to having at home might need to be adjusted on a gastritis diet.

Whether you're preparing meat, eggs, or veggies, it's also important to keep in mind that certain ingredients used for flavor can contribute to irritation. While you might assume you'll want to avoid very spicy foods, there are some ingredients you might not expect to be inflammatory.

Check the ingredients on packaged seasonings, dressings, glazes, or marinades, as they likely contain many spices or herbs. Even relatively basic options like black pepper and garlic can irritate gastritis.

Avoid using large amounts of butter, tomato-based pasta sauce, or rich, creamy, sauces like alfredo when cooking pasta. Try a dash of salt and a drizzle of extra virgin olive oil instead.

Considerations

In addition to the specifics of your gastritis diet plan, you'll want to think about how changing what you eat might affect other areas of your life. When you make changes to your diet, you may also make other adjustments, such as when you're grocery shopping and planning meals for your family, school, and work.

You may also have to pay more attention to how food factors into your social life, such as dining out with friends or attending events where you will need to think about your meal options.

General Nutrition

You'll have many tasty and nutritious options to choose from on the list of approved foods, but there may be some foods you're used to eating that you'll have to reduce or eliminate completely.

Sweets and fast food are tasty and usually OK in moderation, but if you have gastritis avoiding these foods can make a big difference to your symptoms.

You might miss your favorite treats, but french fries, pastries, and fried meat and seafood don't enrich your diet by way of essential vitamins and minerals—so you won't miss them in terms of nutrition. In addition to improving your symptoms and preventing gastritis from getting worse, avoiding heavily processed food that's high in fat, sugar, and salt can also improve your overall health.

Safety

The overall recommendations for a gastritis diet are likely safe for most people, as they aren't overly restrictive. You can also adapt your meal plans if you are following a special diet. If you have gastritis chronically or due to an ongoing medical condition, your doctor might want you to take medication. It's important to tell your doctor about your diet as well as any nutritional supplements you take.

Most medications (whether prescribed or over-the-counter) used to treat gastritis are not likely to interact with foods approved for the diet, but depending on how you adjust the diet to suit your individual tastes and needs, you will want to be aware of the potential for foods and drinks to affect certain drugs.

For example, antacids such as Tums, Rolaids, Mylanta, and Alka-Seltzer may help relieve symptoms of gastritis. Eating calcium-containing foods, such as dairy products or juices enriched with calcium, at the same time as taking an antacid can make them ineffective.3 You should also avoid taking a calcium supplement or vitamin with calcium with an antacid.

Drinking alcohol can also make antacids less effective as well as interact with other medications used to treat gastritis, such as these proton pump inhibitors (PPIs):

- Prilosec
- Nexium
- Prevacid
- Protonix
- Pepcid, a histamine 2 (H2) blocker, is also less effective when combined with alcohol.

These medications reduce the amount of acid in your stomach, while alcohol increases acid production, which can worsen symptoms of gastritis or make the condition worse.

If you have gastritis from infection with H. pylori your doctor may want you to take antibiotics, which interact with a number of foods, drinks, and other medications. You may also need to take antibiotics for another reason while you are also being treated for gastritis. Certain classes of antibiotics interact with medications used to treat gastritis.

While you may not be putting your health at risk, it's best to talk to your doctor before changing your medication or diet if you have gastritis.

Navigating food choices with gastritis is tough. But there are some rules of thumb. Below are some tips for each meal, plus some recipes for added inspiration.

Breakfast

Your best bet in the morning will be a few slices of toast (no butter!) with some slices of banana, or a bowl of oats, again with some banana slices, but with lactose free or low fat milk.

- Add banana, apple and pears to your oats
- Small meals at breakfast and throughout the day are best.
- You can start adding leafy greens like spinach, as well as avocado, and eggs once you can eat grainy toast and oats without pain.
- Try and avoid sweeteners like sugar or honey initially whilst you're in the calming stage.

- Really important to avoid any foods high in grease or fats.That includes bacon, breakfast meats or sausages, or anything fried.
- Sip your water after or before your breakfast, not whilst you're eating
- Stay clear of juices, coffee or tea initially.

Snacks

- Bananas, pears, apples, keep these fruits up
- Try and get in lots of small meals and snacks rather than large meals throughout the day
- Aim for calming but high fibre snacks
- Celery and carrots
- Cranberries are great due to their flavonoid content
- low fat cheeses only once you're stomaching a basic diet (cheddar is good)
- Yoghurt (low in sugar and fat) once you're back on track, will keep your healthy gut thriving
- No chocolate, lollies, soft drinks, bakery goods, packaged foods, cookies, crisps.

Lunch & Dinner

- Brown rice, barley and grainy bread are your staples
- Chicken broth or noodle soup is a great idea in the early days. Add carrot, celery, herbs.
- Lean meats such as turkey and chicken, as well as fish are your go to proteins
- With soups, ensure you don't add high fat creams
- Leafy green veg with all your meals: spinach, rocket,
- If you're vegetarian you can eat Tofu and leafy green veg
- Beans are great, as are broccoli and broccolini
- Then start introducing a bigger range of fibre rich, bright and colourful veggies with your meals as well as lentils and peas, all great fibre rich options for a healthy gut.
- No alcohol!
- Remember, sip water before and after your meal, not with it

- Try and leave a decent amount of time between dinner and bedtime to aid digestion

Conclusions

Gastritis can be painful, but there are some changes you can make that may markedly improve your symptoms and prevent the condition from getting worse. Eating healthy foods and avoiding those that can trigger inflammation, such as those that are fatty or acidic, can both lessen the pain and other symptoms associated with gastritis as well as prevent irritation of the stomach lining from getting worse. Your doctor may also want you to take medications to treat gastritis, but they may not work as well if you include certain foods and drinks in your diet. For the most part, a gastritis diet provides adequate nutrition and can be adapted to suit your unique dietary needs and preferences.

If you are experiencing any symptoms of gastritis, consult a doctor immediately. Untreated gastritis can lead to more medical complications. Following a healthy lifestyle and healthy eating habits plays a major role in alleviating gastrointestinal symptoms. If you struggle with eat healthily, consult a registered dietitian to come up with a diet plan that works for you.

Made in the USA
Las Vegas, NV
08 October 2023